MW01287109

Keto Meal Prep Cookbook:

The Ultimate Ketogenic Meal Prep Guide for Weight Loss and Weight Maintenance.

Includes: Quick and Easy Diet Plan for Beginners. Breakfast, Lunch and Dinner

Table of Contents

Introduction
Chapter 1: Why and How to Meal Prep.................8
Chapter 2: Storing and Rewarming Meals..........20
Chapter 3: Keto Breakfast Recipes......................31
  1. Chicken Maple Sausage Rounds
  2. Avocado Shake
  3. Keto Friendly Toast and Sugarless Jam
  4. Keto Bagels
  5. Omelette Bake
  6. Keto Coffee
  7. Chia and Coconut Bars
  8. Spinach and Bacon Frittata
  9. Cheesy Ham and Broccoli Egg Muffins
  10. Stuffed Breakfast Biscuits
Chapter 4: Keto Lunch Recipes............................57
  1. Pinwheels
  2. No Bun Bacon Burger
  3. Vietnamese Meatballs
  4. Tuna Zucchini Casserole
  5. Hamburger Casserole
  6. Indian Inspired Sloppy Joes
  7. Turkey and Vegetable Stew
  8. Sweet and Sour Pork
  9. Chile Cheese Burgers
  10. Bacon Wrapped Chicken Pepper Bites
Chapter 5: Keto Dinner Recipes............................91
  1. Enchilada Chicken

2. Steak Bits
3. Sausage and Bacon Meatballs
4. Chicken Fajitas
5. Pizza Style Chicken
6. Low Carb Chili
7. Thai Chicken Soup
8. Broccoli Cheese Soup
9. Pork and Pepper Stew
10. Cabbage Lasagna

Bonus Recipe
1. Cloud Bread

Conclusion..123

© Copyright 2018 by Kristian Mckinney - All rights reserved.

The following eBook is reproduced below with the goal of providing information that is as accurate and reliable as possible. Regardless, purchasing this eBook can be seen as consent to the fact that both the publisher and the author of this book are in no way experts on the topics discussed within and that any recommendations or suggestions that are made herein are for entertainment purposes only. Professionals should be consulted as needed prior to undertaking any of the action endorsed herein.

This declaration is deemed fair and valid by both the American Bar Association and the Committee of Publishers Association and is legally binding throughout the United States.

Furthermore, the transmission, duplication or reproduction of any of the following work including specific information will be considered an illegal act irrespective of if it is done electronically or in print. This extends to creating a secondary or tertiary copy of the work or a recorded copy and is only allowed with an expressed written consent from the Publisher. All additional rights reserved.

The information in the following pages is broadly considered to be a truthful and accurate account of facts, and as such any inattention, use or misuse of the information in question by the reader will render any resulting actions solely under their purview. There are no scenarios in which the publisher or the original author of this work can be in any fashion deemed liable for any hardship or damages that may befall them after undertaking information described herein.

Additionally, the information in the following pages is intended only for informational purposes and should thus be thought of as universal. As befitting its nature, it is presented without assurance regarding its prolonged validity or interim quality. Trademarks that are mentioned are done without written consent and can in no way be considered an endorsement from the trademark holder.

Introduction

Congratulations on downloading *Meal Prep for the Keto Diet*. We are excited about your journey as you venture into the world of meal planning in conjunction with your Keto diet. Whether you are new to the lifestyle or a seasoned veteran, this cookbook will provide you with a helpful guide to keeping your culinary life low in carbs and even lower in stress.

The goal of the Ketogenic diet is to stop feeding the body a high concentration of carbohydrates and increase consumption of healthy fats to train the body to burn fat for energy instead of sugars. This is done by sending the body into a metabolic state called ketosis in which fat is turned into energy for the body and brain rather than turning carbohydrates into sugars to be used for energy. Sending the body into a state of ketosis eventually causes the body to burn stored fat. When you start incorporating a Ketogenic diet into your lifestyle, it can be difficult to avoid carbohydrates as they infiltrate so many foods that are consumed in the average diet. Through preparing meals in advance, you allow yourself a full menu of trustworthy foods while saving time and hassle without sacrificing results.

The following chapters will discuss the benefits of meal prepping while on a Ketogenic diet and how to meal prep effectively, as well as including thirty amazing recipes to make your Keto diet practical and sustainable. Each recipe is as detailed as possible, including an estimated prep time, the number of servings and a macronutrient breakdown showing the net carbs, proteins, and fats in each serving. This recipe compilation provides options to help you satisfy your cravings without ditching your diet, as well as adding variety to your meal plan.

There are plenty of books on meal prepping and the Ketogenic diet on the market, so thank you for choosing this one! We've worked hard to provide you with the most helpful guide possible, and we hope you enjoy!

Short positive review on Amazon is always much appreciated ☺

Chapter 1: Why and How-to Meal Prep

Implementing lifestyle changes is difficult, especially when life has a habit of moving quickly. Avoiding carbs seems like a simple idea until it's the middle of the week, there's work to be done and buying a sandwich from the deli down the street is much easier to fit into your schedule than cooking a diet-approved gourmet lunch. Preparing meals ahead of time allows you to save time and money on cooking, as well as the added benefit of knowing what's going into your food.

Let's start with a look into what the Ketogenic diet entails to further allow understanding of why meal prep will fit well into your Keto life. The overall goal of this diet is to reach a metabolic state of ketosis. When the body is in a state of ketosis, the energy for the brain and body is coming from fats rather than sugars. Normally, our body gets energy from sugars in the form of glucose. When the body is fed carbohydrates, the carbs are processed into sugars. As the body reaches capacity for the amount of sugar it needs to function, the carbohydrates begin to be stored as fat. The Keto diet follows the macronutrient contents of food to determine which foods to consume and in what quantities. A standard Keto diet allows approximately 5 percent of the consumption for the day to be of carbohydrates. Approximately 20 percent of the calories consumed on the diet consists of proteins, and the large majority of the diet is made up of fats which fill out the other 75 percent of the contents. By avoiding carbohydrates and sugars in a strict manner, the body no longer has this source for energy, so it looks elsewhere. This energy is found in ketone bodies which are created by the liver from breaking down fats. This is why the Keto diet focuses heavily on consuming healthy fats to provide ketones that are used to fuel the body. Because the body is utilizing fat for energy, it will also start burning stored fat. Glucose will still be present in the body, but in much smaller quantities. By a process called gluconeogenesis, things other than carbohydrates are turned into glucose. Protein can be turned into glucose to maintain healthy levels in the blood. There are also some tissues in the body that are not able to be fueled by ketones. Red blood cells and some parts of the brain need glucose to function. This is why gluconeogenesis is important, although some people are concerned that it will cause too much glucose production and kick the body out of ketosis. This is not very likely, but if it is something you are concerned about then be aware of what products fuel the process and to what extent.

This lifestyle is an effective way to lose weight and get healthier. It has been shown to help in improving the lives of people living with type 2 diabetes as it lowers the levels of insulin production. It has also been proven to lessen the frequency of uncontrolled seizures in children with epileptic episodes. This use was the original application for the diet. Keto has also shown promise in cancer patients, although these claims are not as well substantiated. Overall, there is a large belief that the benefits of Keto range far beyond simple fat loss. During a duration of approximately one week after beginning the Keto diet, people may experience a state called "Keto flu." This occurs when the body is not receiving the fuel it is accustomed to but has not yet realized that it should begin finding fuel elsewhere. Symptoms may include discomfort in the gastrointestinal tract, nausea, irritability, and brain fog. However, after the body has become accustomed to its new diet, mental clarity and mood may prove to be better than on a normal diet. Some people find that the clarity of their skin improves, and their sleep is more restful, as well as finding that they're losing fat while still feeling more satiated by their meals. Experience varies from person to person, but many people enjoy the benefits of a Keto diet in one way or another. One of the bigger downsides of this diet is that many people find it difficult to maintain. Avoiding pasta, bread, beer, grains and sugary foods as well as not being able to consume fruits or even potatoes severely narrows down the available food. If you are trying to follow a Keto diet during a busy week, it can be difficult to find time to cook proper food, and the available alternatives are slim. There are many Keto substitutes for the foods you'll avoid on the diet, so you won't generally have to go without. These substitutes are also usually made on your own, so you can be confident about the ingredients they contain. By utilizing meal prep tactics, you provide yourself with the opportunity to have food available that suits your diet and allows you to continue practicing this lifestyle.

Meal prepping takes a little investment, but the rewards to be reaped make it well worthwhile. A weekend afternoon can be spent cooking multiple meals that will easily store in the refrigerator or freezer until they're needed. When it's time to eat, simply remove the meal from cold storage, reheat and enjoy! The process is a little time consuming, but fairly straightforward, and this book is a great resource to help you get started. The first step is to decide what meals you plan to eat throughout the week. Once you've chosen, collect the ingredients for all of the meals. Eating the same food for multiple meals will make meal prepping much easier as you can make larger quantities of the same thing rather than making different foods. Along the same line, eating different meals with the same ingredients can allow a bit more variety and still save time. For instance, if you would like to eat two different meals that involve riced cauliflower, you can double the amount of cauliflower that you are preparing ahead of time and use it in different ways. Once your ingredients are ready, prepare all of your meals for the week and store as desired. Your future self will be grateful!

When following a Keto diet, planning meals ahead of time will reduce stress throughout the week and ensure that you have an easier time sticking to the prescribed foods. When choosing meals, knowing what foods you tend to crave or which high carb meals you miss eating can be key in staying on track with your keto diet. Find a diet-approved alternative and incorporate it into your meal plan! Think about what meals you would like to eat in the upcoming week and form a grocery list of low carb ingredients and healthy fats. If you choose meals with similar ingredients, such as a lunch and a dinner that both include chicken, this can help cut down on both cost and prep time. The drawback of this hack is that eating only the same foods can get dull and cause demotivation to stick to a diet. While you'll want to be sure to incorporate enough variety to stay on track, don't over complicate your meal prep. Trying to prepare multiple intricate meals in one afternoon will be time-consuming and can leave you feeling uninspired to meal prep in the following weeks. Find a balance that works for you and plan your meals accordingly.

 Once your food is prepared, you will need containers to freeze or refrigerate the food. What type of containers you use will depend on which method of meal prepping you decide is best for you. Some people find that simply preparing ingredients ahead of time so that minimal effort is needed when putting together a meal takes some of the stress away and still feels like a freshly cooked meal. If you're looking to pack lunches for work or need meals you can eat on the go, you may want to go the route of individually portioning meals. Maybe you don't have time to prepare meals during the week, but you also don't have space in your refrigerator or freezer for 21 individually packaged meals. In that case, you can store pre-cooked meals like a casserole in the icebox and portion them out as you go. Perhaps you come across a weekend where you have some extra time, and you'd like to prepare extra food to be frozen and used over the next couple of months. With a method called "batch cooking," you can prepare large quantities of food and utilize them over an extended period of time. For instance, you may prepare more Keto friendly sausages (recipe here) than you need for one week. This is a perfect time to portion out your upcoming breakfasts and pop the extra sausages in the freezer for your future self to enjoy.

Individual portioning is an increasingly popular method of preparing meals in advance. It's a fairly straightforward process; a full, balanced meal is prepared and separated into containers, then refrigerated or frozen so you don't have to worry about squeezing any food preparation time into your busy schedule later in the week. Pre-portioning meals is an ideal choice when following a diet, like Keto, that involves meeting certain quantities of macronutrients like fats, proteins and carbs as you can measure out how much of each food you need for a complete meal, place it all in one convenient container and cut out the guesswork of trying to calculate servings later on. Any type of food storage container can be used, but keep in mind that when freezers and microwaves are involved, you want to be sure your dish is suitable for the task. This may also be a tough method to implement if you're low on space, so you'll want to make sure your containers aren't too large. Each meal is placed in a separate container so you can imagine how that starts to add up when you're preparing meals for a week in advance. Some people find it helpful to combine this meal prep method with others by individually portioning specific meals for busier parts of the day, like a grab-and-go lunch to take to work but using other meal prep methods for meals that don't need to be as readily available.

When you're running low on fridge space but want to have a meal prepared, a make-ahead meal like casserole or soup may be the fit for you. With this method, the meal is fully cooked and stored for later reheating, but it isn't separated into portions. This may also be a great way to prepare when you're going to be serving multiple people. It's up to you if you want to store your make-ahead meal in the same dish in which it was cooked or transfer it to another, just keep in mind that any container used for cold storage should be freezer safe.

When preparing meals, you greatly enjoy, it can be helpful to cook larger quantities and use them over a longer period of time. This method is called batch cooking and can be very useful when it comes to foods that are consumed more frequently. In the winter months, a food like this low-carb, keto chili may become a staple. Doubling the batch can yield results for a week's meals while also providing plenty to be saved for a cold night when the chili craving hits. Batch cooking also allows you to save money. When making large quantities of food, the ingredients can be purchased in bulk. Generally, the more you buy of a product, the less you pay for each unit of that product. This cost-effective perk can be attributed to meal prepping as a whole.

As helpful and time-saving as rewarming pre-cooked meals can be, sometimes it's not ideal. Meal prepping techniques can still be used to make your culinary life more manageable. Preparing individual ingredients that are used frequently can save time and reduce stress. Pre-ricing cauliflower, mincing garlic or mixing sauces removes a few time-consuming steps from later meal preparation. In the keto lifestyle, home mixed seasonings and sauces are regularly substituted in lieu of processed and carb heavy store-bought options. Preparing these ahead of time can help to keep your diet on track as well as being easier on your wallet and your schedule.

Sticking to any singular method of meal prep is not always practical when you lead a busy life. Preparing a few pre-portioned meals for workday lunch breaks or quick morning breakfasts while also having a pot of soup or a casserole for evening meals will save storage space. Leaving a few meals uncooked may break the monotony of eating already cooked meals. The ingredients for these can be prepared ahead of time during your meal prep day so when the time comes your meal will be easy and satisfying to assemble. There is no universal system that you are required to use when your meal prep. Experiment and find what suits your needs. Keep in mind that as your life changes, your meal prep may need to adapt as well. Family visiting from out of town may be a reason to prepare a make-ahead meal such as a casserole, while longer work days may require a larger quantity of pre-portioned meals. The great thing about this lifestyle choice is that it puts you in control of your meals and can be easily tailored to your specific needs.

While you are cooking, you may try to multitask. If you want to make two recipes that are baked at the same temperature and your oven can accommodate both pans, try cooking both at the same time. Be sure to pay attention to the cook time for each recipe. Setting a timer can help to make multitasking more possible. If you're worried that you won't be able to safely bake two meals at once, that's not a problem. Other small multitasking hacks can still help you. If one recipe calls for a longer baking or simmering time, choose a recipe to prep the same day that can be prepared while you wait. The fajita chicken recipe in chapter 5 needs to bake for a duration of 20 to 25 minutes once it is assembled. During this time, the pinwheels mentioned in chapter 4 can easily be made in 15 minutes. Taking preparation time into account when scheduling your meals and prep days can help you use your time efficiently and make the process a little less frustrating.

Many foods that are used to make the recipes in this book are staples for keto meals. Knowing which staple foods, you will need can help you to save money. Knowing that many Keto meals contain avocado because it is high in healthy fats may encourage you to stock up on avocados when well-ripened options are available. See chapter 2 for a few tips on how to freeze avocados for later use so you won't have to throw them out if you don't get around to using them right away. Other staple ingredients include eggs, chicken, almond flour and coconut oil. Many other ingredients could also be considered staples for the keto diet, but these specifically are common throughout this cookbook. Purchasing larger quantities of ingredients that are used commonly can reduce the price per unit. Non-perishable items can be stored for extended periods of time without decreasing their quality.

Understanding meal prep is generally very simple. In fact, simplicity is one of the key ingredients to a successful meal prep lifestyle. Planning ahead will change everything. Plan what meals you want to make, make a list of the groceries you will need to accomplish that, plan the preparation and cook times for the meals to coincide, and plan the space you will use to store the food. Don't try to overload yourself with making difficult meals all in one afternoon and don't choose meals that you know will not be appealing more than once.

Chapter 2: Storing and Rewarming Meals

One aspect of meal prepping that will help you have the most satisfying meals possible is ensuring that prepared foods are properly stored and reheated to maintain their ideal flavors and textures. Some foods can be frozen and thawed without losing their pizzazz, while others may only be able to hold up in the refrigerator for a couple of days. Knowing which foods can be prepared in large batches and used over time will help you save time and can help when choosing staple meals, while some foods that only keep a few days can still be prepared at the beginning of any given week to allow for variety.

When storing prepared foods, it is highly important to ensure you have the proper container for the job. Freezer and microwave-safe containers are ideal, and dishwasher-safe is an added bonus. Glass containers are much easier to clean and tend to hold up longer without staining. However, a plastic container may be sufficient, it's up to you to decide. It is also important to be certain that all food storage containers have a tightly sealing lid that will help maintain freshness. Poorly sealed foods can get soggy and stale, which may make it difficult to stick to your diet rather than tossing your prepared meal for something more appetizing. Also, pay attention to the temperature of your refrigerator and freezer. To keep food stored at an ideal temperature, a refrigerator should be colder than 35 degrees Fahrenheit, and a freezer should be colder than zero degrees Fahrenheit.

If you're preparing individually portioned meals, it may be ideal to purchase food storage containers with separate sections that can increase the ease of portioning different foods. A larger container may lead you to portion larger servings, if you're not careful, which could lead to overeating and wastefulness. A too small container may prevent proper portioning, causing too little food to be packed which can leave you with a meal that is unsatisfactory in size, or insufficient in macros. However, a well-selected container will hold the proper amount of food for a balanced meal and will appear fuller than a too large container. This allows your brain to avoid feeling that you are being served inadequate portion sizes and will leave you more likely to feel satiated after your meal. Measuring one serving of each food into the container will help you ensure that you are aware of the macro count in each meal. As you can tell, finding the right food containers is a crucial step toward a successful meal prep, and it depends deeply on what best suits your lifestyle.

After your meals have been stored, many will need to be rewarmed before it's time to eat. Meals with different base ingredients will need to be reheated in different ways to ensure they maintain as much of their flavor and texture as possible. When planning meals, it is important to know how to preserve the integrity of your food so that you can get maximum enjoyment out of your meal. This will help you decide which foods to freeze and which to refrigerate, as well as knowing how to properly cook each food for reheating.

Many meat-based meals, such as these steak bits, store well in the freezer and reheat without losing their flavor and feel. If properly stored, meatballs and sausages can be stored in the freezer for up to 3 months without losing their quality. Allow frozen foods to thaw before reheating. The best way to do this is to place the frozen goods in the refrigerator the night before. This allows the food's temperature to rise slowly and evens out the thawing. Placing frozen goods on the counter to thaw can cause the food to reach, and stay at, room temperature which can begin allowing bacteria to breed over time. If you're on the go, removing a pre-prepared meal from the freezer in the morning before work and taking it with you should allow it to thaw enough by lunchtime that it can be reheated easily. While this is less ideal than defrosting in the refrigerator, the food should not thaw to a concerning temperature during a short time, and if you ensure the food is heated to a proper temperature before being eaten, you shouldn't have to worry.

When reheating meats, it is again ideal to thaw them in the refrigerator beforehand. If the time for this is lacking, place the meat in a water-tight plastic bag and hold it under a stream of cold water. The more thawed your meat is before being heated, the faster it will reach the desired temperature. This prevents any excess cooking of the food. It is important to be aware that some meats tend to dry out when reheated. When using a microwave, cutting dryer meats like chicken into smaller pieces will allow them to heat faster and reduce the risk of being parched. Placing a damp paper towel over the plate can help to keep the meat moist. Opting for a stovetop may be more ideal for foods like steak or chicken breast. Adding a pad of grass-fed butter or a tablespoon of coconut oil to the meat as it warms can lend a bit of moisture and also incorporate some healthy, Keto friendly fats! This is also a helpful tip if an oven is being used. Set the oven to a low temperature and place the food inside with your choice of fatty addition. This method takes longer but preserves the integrity of your foods flavor and texture better than other methods.

Meals with sautéed vegetables will also need a bit of water or a damp paper towel in the microwave to allow them to heat through steaming. If you prepare the vegetables with the intention of reheating them for later consumption, it may be helpful to leave them slightly undercooked. This reduces the risk of overcooking during the rewarming process. Once again, it is important to remember to thaw frozen foods before attempting to reheat them. If your vegetables are part of a dish that includes meat or other ingredients, note the different durations needed to reach the ideal temperature. It may be best to heat ingredients separately if the opportunity is available. If this is not possible or you wish to save the time, be sure to stir the food occasionally during the process to allow even warming. Using a pan over a stovetop is a better option for vegetables than the microwave. Add a bit of oil (yay, healthy fats!) and stir as they heat. The oven is less ideal, but if you'd like to warm vegetables this way, be sure to use a low heat and add some oil to keep them a little crisper.

Soups and casseroles are a little trickier to reheat. When being prepared, it is best to leave the dish slightly undercooked, so the integrity of the meal is not compromised in the reheating process. Both casseroles and soups can be frozen for up to 3 months. Casseroles are best reheated in the oven at a medium temperature for a duration of 20 to

30 minutes. If you do not wish to reheat the entirety of the dish, a single portion can be warmed in the microwave. Note that this method will be more likely to leave your food watery. If the casserole contains a larger amount of vegetables, there may also be excess water when it is thawed from frozen. If possible, drain excess water before warming. Be sure to heat the food to a high temperature. This may require cooking it longer and waiting for the food to cool before consumption. Casseroles do not reheat well on a stovetop, so this method is not recommended. If this is the only method available to you, add some water or oil to a lidded pot to ensure the food does not dry out. Soups present the opposite problem. Ingredients can lose texture due to the moisture of the soup. Depending on the ingredients of the soup, this can alter how you prepare and heat it. When vegetables are involved, it is best to leave the soup slightly undercooked so that the vegetables do not become soggy when it's time to eat. As always, thaw food before warming. When reheating, it's naturally ideal to bring the pot to a boil over the stove. Be sure to leave space at the top of the pot to avoid any unexpected mess. Soups containing dairy products should be heated slowly over a medium to high heat to avoid curdling. When using a microwave, be sure to use a dish that allows room at the top for expansion during

heating. Place the food into the microwave for increments of 30 seconds, stirring between, until soup is very hot. Allow it to cool before eating.

Cooked eggs can be frozen for a duration of up to 6 months, but it is best to eat them before 3 months has passed. Frozen eggs will maintain their best consistency if they are whipped before being cooked. The egg recipes in this cookbook all involve beating the eggs prior to frying or baking so they will freeze and reheat easily. An oven is the best way to warm frozen eggs as it will be less likely to leave them rubbery. A duration of 12 to 15 minutes on a medium heat should thoroughly heat the eggs. If you want a quicker method, a microwave will work fine. Place the frozen eggs into the microwave for a duration of 5 to 7 minutes. Be aware of how other ingredients in breakfast foods need to be warmed and choose a method accordingly.

Ensure that when you plan your meals, you are aware of how to reheat them. This can affect how they are stored, whether they are frozen or refrigerated, and which foods are paired together. Plates with different types of foods can be reheated without separating their contents. In situations like this, it is important to mix the food as it cooks to ensure even warming and prevent some ingredients from getting overdone during the process. This is especially important when dealing with meals containing water-retaining vegetables that have been frozen. If foods are being microwaved, particularly when food is being heated to very high temperatures, be sure to use a dish that is suitable for the job. Microwaving plastic wrap is not ideal unless it is specifically designed for the task. Microwaving plastic containers may also be less than ideal. This is because plastic can melt and contaminate the food. If you do wish to use a plastic container, be sure it is BPA free.

Some pre-prepared meals will not require warming. A breakfast shake like the one mentioned in Chapter 3 can be prepped in various ways. The shake can be fully blended and refrigerated to be consumed in a matter one or two days, or the blended shake can be frozen and thawed when it's time to consume. The thawing may change the texture and could be less ideal. The ingredients for the shake can also be assembled in a plastic bag or jar to be placed in the freezer, and when you're ready, the bag can be emptied into a blender with a little water. Choose a method of preparation that suits your needs. Keto Coffee is also a recipe that may not necessarily be rewarmed. In the same way, as the avocado shake can be portioned and assembled later, ingredients for Keto Coffee can be frozen separately and then added together to a small plastic bag in individual portions. When you are ready to add the healthy fats to your fresh, hot coffee and blend, empty one bag containing a portion of each fat into the cup.

Low-carb bread should be stored in the refrigerator. Some breads can be frozen. If you want to freeze the bread, add it to an airtight plastic bag before adding it to the freezer. When ready to consume, there are three ways to defrost your bread. If you are looking to make toast, just add the frozen bread to the toaster. The duration of toasting will increase by 1 to 2 minutes. For other uses, add the bread to the microwave for a duration of 15 to 20 seconds at a high power. This will soften the bread. Be sure to add the bread when it is frozen and ensure you have not let it thaw beforehand. Another method of defrosting bread is to add the bread to a baking sheet then add the baking sheet to an oven that is set to a temperature of 325 degrees Fahrenheit for a duration of approximately 5 minutes.

Avocados can be frozen for a duration of up to 6 months. Once thawed, these avocados will not be ideal for use in slices or as a topping for other foods, but they can be used in smoothies or dressings afterward. There are a few ways to freeze avocado. You can cut the avocado in half and take out the seed before peeling the skin. It's important to ensure that you add lemon juice or lime juice to both sides of the avocado halves so you will not end up with brown goo. After you add the lemon juice, add the halves to a plastic bag and make sure to take out as much air as possible. To get very tightly wrapped halves, you can use plastic wrap if you wish, but ensure the avocado is well wrapped. If you want to fill the plastic bags more and ensure the avocado is less likely to become brown, the halves can be cut into smaller pieces. Add the pieces to a bowl and add 2 teaspoons of lemon juice to the bowl for each large avocado. You can fit more avocado into each bag with this method. The best method to freeze avocados for avocado smoothies is to mash them before adding them to the freezer. This will ensure a smoother blend after the frozen avocado is thawed. Using a blender or food processor can blend the avocado more effectively before freezing. If this is not available to you, you can just use a regular fork. Be sure to add lemon juice in the same quantity as other methods as you puree the fruit. The puree can be added to ice cube trays or to plastic bags. To thaw frozen avocados, add them to the refrigerator overnight or for a number of hours before you want to use them. Alternatively, frozen avo can be added to a counter for a duration of approximately one hour to thaw at room temperature. If you need the avocado quickly, add one whole avocado's worth of frozen avo to the microwave for a duration of less than one minute.

Chapter 3: Keto Breakfast Recipes

When following a keto diet, it can be easy to fall into a routine of bacon and eggs for every breakfast. While using such a delicious combination as a staple meal is not a bad thing, here is a compilation of ten morning meals low in carbohydrates and high in flavor to add variety.

Chicken Maple Sausage Rounds

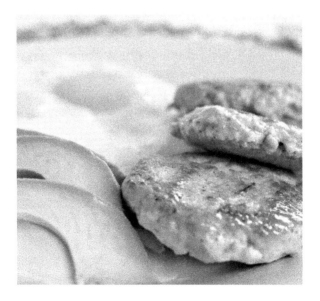

This recipe needs 20 minutes to prepare and makes 8 portions.

One portion size is 2 rounds; it contains:

11 grams Fat

21 grams Protein

1.4 grams Carbs

187 Calories

What's in It

- Ground Cloves (pinch)
- Ground Nutmeg (.25 teaspoons)
- Red Pepper Flakes (.25 teaspoons)
- Dry Thyme (.5 teaspoons)
- Black Pepper (1 teaspoon)
- Onion Powder (1 teaspoon)
- Garlic Powder (1 teaspoon)
- Dry Parsley (1.5 teaspoons)
- Sage (2 teaspoons)
- Pink Salt (2 teaspoons)
- Sugarless Maple Syrup (3 tablespoons)
- *Minced* Chicken (2 pounds)
- Oil (1 tablespoon)

Also Needed

- Large Mixing Bowl
- Frying Pan

How It's Made

- All contents except oil should be well combined in the bowl before being shaped into round patties that each contain 2 ounces of the mixture.
- Add the pan to the stove over a burner that is turned to medium heat before adding 1 tablespoon of oil to the pan.
- Allow the oil to heat before adding meat to the pan until each side is brown and the patties are cooked thoroughly.
- Before placing the cooked sausage in a container for later consumption, remove patties from the pan and allow to cool.

Note

This recipe can be changed a few ways. The patties can be baked rather than fried in a skillet. Cooked patties will freeze well, as will uncooked patties. Form the sausages and freeze them on parchment paper until the patties are solid. Then place the frozen patties in an airtight container until you are ready for them. For tips on storing and rewarming meat see here.

Avocado Shake

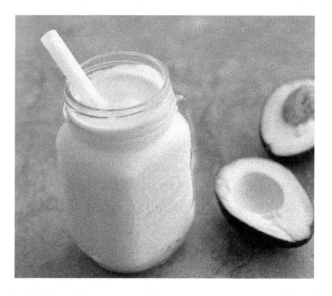

This recipe needs 5 minutes to prepare and makes 2 portions.

One portion size is 1 pint; it contains:

43 grams Fat

8 grams Protein

20 grams Carbs

491 Calories

What's in It

- Strawberries (.25 cups)
- Cinnamon (.25 teaspoons)
- Cream of Coconut (2 cups)
- Mint (.5 cup chopped)
- Avocado (.5)

Also Needed:

- Blender
- 2 Glass Jars

How It's Made

- Ensure that the seed and skin are removed from the avocado before adding the avocado to the blender.
- Before adding mint to the blender, cut it into smaller pieces dependent on the necessary size for effective blending.
- Before blending on a high setting for a duration of 30 to 60 seconds, add all remaining contents to the blender.
- Two glass jars can be filled with the shake and kept in a refrigerator for breakfasts.

Note

This recipe can be changed a few ways. The contents of the smoothie besides the cream of coconut can be pre-portioned before being added to a plastic bag and frozen. When ready to be consumed, add the contents of the bag and the coconut cream to the blender. Avocado can be blended before being added to the freezer to ensure a less chunky smoothie. This process is explained here.

Keto Friendly Toast and Sugarless Jam

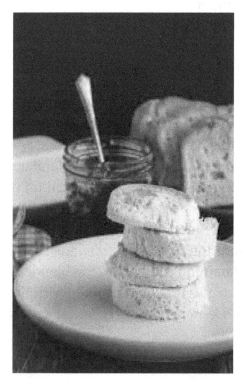

This recipe needs 20 minutes to prepare and makes 4 portions.

One portion size is 2 slices toast with 2 tablespoons of jam; it contains:

17 grams Fat

13 grams Protein

17 grams Carbs

391 Calories

What's in It

Sugarless Jam:
- Chia Seeds (2 tablespoon ground)
- Erythritol (2 tablespoons)
- Juice of Lemon (3 tablespoons)
- Strawberries (2 cups)

Bread:
- Butter (2 tablespoons)
- Baking Powder (1 teaspoon)
- Egg (2 large)
- Almond Flour (.5 cups)
- Coconut Flour (2 tablespoons)

Also Needed:

- Potato Masher or Fork
- Saucepan

- Large Mug

How It's Made

Sugarless Jam:
- Before smashing strawberries with a mashing utensil, add strawberries to a saucepan.
- Before adding the saucepan to the stove above a burner set to a high heat, mix in lemon juice and chia seeds.
- After the saucepan has reached a boil, lessen heat to allow the mixture to simmer for a duration of 60 seconds.
- Before pouring jam into jars, add Erythritol sweetener and allow mixture to cool away from the stove.

Bread:
- Before placing a large mug into the microwave for a duration of 2 minutes, add contents and use a fork to mix all ingredients thoroughly.
- When cooking is completed, remove from mug and slice. Keep in a refrigerator for later consumption.

Note

The jam recipe may make more jam than can be consumed with this amount of bread. Any extra jam should be kept in the refrigerator in a jar. Glass jars will be easiest to clean after the jam is consumed.

Keto Bagels

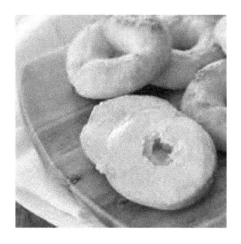

This recipe needs 30 minutes to prepare and cook and makes 6 portions.

One portion size is 1 bagel; it contains:

35.5 grams Fat

27.8 grams Protein

8 grams Carbs

449 Calories

What's in It

- Cream Cheese (5 tablespoons)
- Low Moisture Mozzarella (3 cups shredded)
- Eggs (3 large divided)
- Italian Seasoning (1 teaspoon)
- Onion Powder (1 teaspoon)
- Garlic Powder (1 teaspoon)
- Baking Powder (1 tablespoon)
- Almond Flour (2 cups)

Also Needed:

- Baking Sheet
- Parchment Paper
- Small Bowl
- Large Mixing Bowl

How It's Made

- Before preheating the oven to 425 degrees Fahrenheit, add parchment paper to a baking sheet.
- Add Italian seasoning, onion powder, garlic powder, baking powder and almond flour to a medium sized bowl and mix well.
- Before setting one egg aside, crack it into a small bowl and whisk.

- Add mozzarella and cream cheese to a large bowl before microwaving for a duration of 90 seconds. Microwave for a duration of 60 seconds more after stirring, then stir again.
- Add flour combination to the bowl along with 2 eggs and mix well.
- Split and roll dough into 6 balls before using your finger to create a hole in the middle of each and stretch to form a ring.
- Before adding the baking sheet to oven for a duration of 12-14 minutes, use the whisked egg to brush over top of each ring.
- Bagels can be wrapped in plastic wrap and refrigerated after being removed from oven and cooled.

Note

This recipe can be frozen for later consumption. Learn how frozen bread products can be thawed here.

Omelette Bake

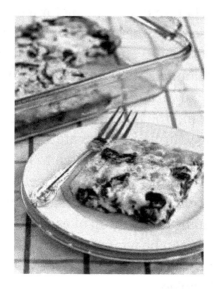

This recipe needs 30 minutes to prepare and cook and makes 6 portions.

One portion size is 1 section; it contains:

11 grams Fat

15 grams Protein

5 grams Carbs

175 Calories

What's in It

- Salt and Pepper (to taste)

- Oregano (.5 teaspoons)
- Feta Cheese (.5 cup)
- Sun-Dried Tomatoes (.25 cup)
- Kale (1 cup chopped)
- Eggs (12 large)

Also Needed:

- Baking Pan
- Foil
- Mixing Bowl

How It's Made

- Ensure that the oven is preheated to a temperature of 350 degrees Fahrenheit.
- Before adding in seasonings, feta cheese, kale, and tomatoes, whisk together eggs in a big bowl.
- Ensure that the baking pan is lined with foil and sprayed with non-stick oil.
- Pour the mixture into the baking pan and add to the oven for a duration of 25 minutes.
- After allowing the omelet bake to cool, portions can be kept in a refrigerator for up to 5 days or frozen for later rewarming.

Note

Cooked eggs can be frozen for a duration of up to 6 months. Ensure the meal has cooled well before freezing. For storage and rewarming instructions, see here.

Keto Coffee

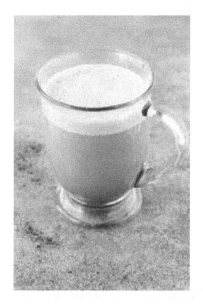

This recipe needs 10 minutes to prepare and makes 4 portions.

One portion size is 1 cup; it contains:

27.7 grams Fat

1.08 grams Protein

1.05 grams Carbs

260 Calories

What's in It

- Vanilla Extract (2 teaspoons)
- Full Cream (2 tablespoons)
- Coconut Oil (4 tablespoons)
- Grass Fed Butter (4 tablespoons)
- Coffee (4 cups brewed)

Also Needed:

- Ice Cube Tray
- Blender

How It's Made

- Ensure you have 1 ice cube tray with a minimum of 12 sections.
- Add vanilla to cream and mix thoroughly before dividing mixture into 4 sections of the ice cube tray.
- Bring butter and coconut oil to a fluid state before dividing into remaining sections. This will make 4 sections coconut oil, 4 sections butter and 4 sections vanilla cream. Add to the freezer.
- Make 4 cups of coffee and add them to a large pourable container in a refrigerator.

- To use prepared ingredients, add 1 cup coffee and 1 cube each of oil, butter and vanilla cream to a blender and mix until frothy.

Note

When using the recipe as a meal prep, coffee can be left out. The oil, butter and vanilla cream cubes can be added to freshly brewed hot coffee on the day in which they are desired to be consumed. To find tips on making pre-portioned keto coffee pouches, see here.

Chia and Coconut Bars

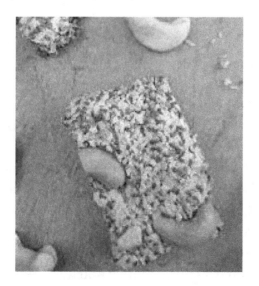

This recipe needs 1 hour to prepare and cook and makes 6 portions.

One portion size is 1 bar; it contains:

14 grams Fat

4 grams Protein

3.5 grams Carbs

164 Calories

What's in It

- Cashews (.5 cups)
- Vanilla Extract (.25 teaspoons)
- Powdered Erythritol (1 teaspoon)
- Coconut Oil (1 tablespoon)
- Unsweetened Coconut Meat (1 cup shredded, dried)
- Water (.5 cup)
- Chia Seeds (4 tablespoons)

Also Needed:

- Medium Bowl
- Baking Pan
- Parchment Paper

How It's Made

- Ensure that baking pan is lined with parchment paper and oven is preheated to a temperature of 350 degrees Fahrenheit.
- Add .5 cups of water to chia seeds in a bowl. After 15 minutes have passed and chia seeds are of a gooey consistency, add vanilla, erythritol, coconut oil and coconut to the bowl and mix well. Add cashews last and mix.
- Before adding the pan to the oven for a duration of 45 minutes, spread the mixture into the pan and flatten.
- Divide cooled result into 6 portions and add to the refrigerator after coating them in plastic wrap.

Spinach and Bacon Frittata

This recipe needs 35 minutes to prepare and makes 4 portions.

One portion size is 1 cup; it contains:

32.3 grams Fat

28.7 grams Protein

4.2 grams Carbs

419 Calories

What's in It

- Black Pepper (.13 teaspoons)
- Sea Salt (.13 teaspoons)
- Spinach (4 cups chopped)
- Bacon (6 slices chopped)
- Coconut Milk (.5 cups)
- Eggs (12 large)

Also Needed:

- Mixing Bowl
- Muffin Tin
- Frying Pan

How It's Made

- Ensure the oven is heated to a temperature of 350 degrees Fahrenheit.
- Add the coconut milk and eggs to a large bowl and whisk.
- Add the pan to a stove above a burner that is set to a medium heat before adding the bacon to the pan and cooking it until it is nearly crisp.
- Before adding the spinach to the pan containing the remaining bacon fat and

cooking until it is wilted, remove the cooked bacon pieces.

- Add spinach to the bowl of egg mixture and mix before pouring the contents into 4 sections of the muffin pan. Drop pieces of bacon on top of each section and add the pan to the oven for a duration of 15 to 20 minutes.

Note

Cooked eggs can be frozen for a duration of up to 6 months. Ensure the meal has cooled well before freezing. For storage and rewarming instructions, see here.

Cheesy Ham and Broccoli Egg Muffins

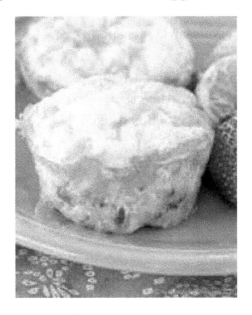

This recipe needs 37 minutes to prepare and makes 12 portions.

One portion size is 1 muffin; it contains:

7 grams Fat

9 grams Protein

1 grams Carbs

115 Calories

What's in It

- Black Pepper (.25 teaspoons)
- Salt (1 teaspoon)
- Dry Mustard (1 teaspoon)
- Eggs (12)
- Cheddar Cheese (4 ounces shredded)
- Ham (1 cup diced)
- Broccoli (1.5 cups cooked)

Also Needed:

- Mixing Bowl
- Muffin Tin

How It's Made

- Ensure the oven is heated to a temperature of 350 degrees Fahrenheit and the muffin tin is lightly coated with oil.
- Add broccoli and ham to each cup of the muffin tin before adding cheddar cheese on top of each. Divide contents equally.
- Add pepper, salt, dry mustard and eggs to a bowl and whip together.
- Add .25 cups of egg mixture to each cup of the muffin tin before adding the muffin tin to the oven for a duration of 20 to 25 minutes.
- Allow results to cool before wrapping in plastic wrap and adding to the freezer.

Note

Cooked eggs can be frozen for a duration of up to 6 months. Ensure the meal has cooled well before freezing. For storage and rewarming instructions, see here.

Stuffed Breakfast Biscuits

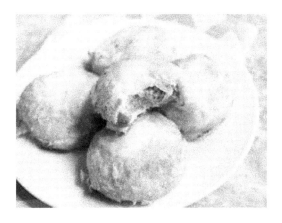

This recipe needs 20 minutes to prepare and makes 6 portions.

One portion size is 1 biscuit; it contains approximately:

20 grams Fat

12 grams Protein

2 grams Carbs

250 Calories

What's in It

- Sausage Patties (6 pre-cooked)
- Colby Jack Cheese (2 ounces cubed)
- Salt (.13 teaspoons)
- Pepper (.13 teaspoons)
- Almond Flour (1 cup)
- Eggs (2 beaten)
- Mozzarella Cheese (2 cups shredded)
- Cream Cheese (2 ounces)

Also Needed:

- Bowl (2 small)
- Muffin Tin

How It's Made

- Ensure the oven is heated to a temperature of 400 degrees Fahrenheit and a muffin tin is lightly oiled.
- Add the mozzarella cheese and cream cheese to a bowl before adding the bowl to a microwave for a duration of 30 seconds.
- Take the bowl out of the microwave and stir well before adding the bowl into the

microwave again for a duration of 30 seconds.

- Repeat this process until the mozzarella cheese is melting and the cream cheese is very soft. Ensure the cheeses are well mixed.
- Add the almond flour and eggs to an empty bowl to mix before adding the cheese mix to the flour and eggs.
- Add a dusting of almond flour to the dough and make a ball before adding the dough to the refrigerator until it is firm.
- Separate the firm dough into 6 balls that are each approximately 3 inches wide.
- Press each ball of dough so that it is flat.
- Add one piece of cheese and one sausage to each flattened piece of dough.
- Wrap the dough around the sausage and cheese before placing each into one section of the muffin tin.
- Add the muffin tin to the oven for a duration of 12 to 15 minutes.
- Ensure biscuits are cooled thoroughly before adding them to the freezer. Microwave for a duration of 1 minute before eating.

Note

These stuffed biscuits will freeze well and may be consumed for up to a week after preparation. This dough recipe can also be used to make biscuits that are not stuffed for to substitute for other recipes when you want a bread-like option.

Chapter 4: Keto Lunch Recipes

Life gets busy and figuring out what to eat on your lunch break each day can take away precious time you could use for more important things. These lunch choices are easily prepared ahead of time and can allow you to savor your saved time just as much as you'll savor this food. Freeze certain meals, and when you take them out of the freezer in the morning, they will thaw just enough to be reheated when it's time for lunch.

Pinwheels

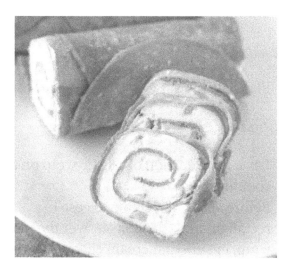

This recipe needs 15 minutes to prepare and makes 20 portions.

One portion size is 2 wheels; it contains:

7.5 grams Fat

2 grams Protein

2 grams Carbs

94 Calories

What's in It

- Pickles (4 tablespoons diced)
- Genoa Salami (6 large thin slices)
- Pepperoni (6 large thin slices)
- Cream Cheese (8 ounces)

Also Needed:

- Plastic Wrap

How It's Made

- Lay a large section of plastic wrap on the counter.
- Before spreading cream cheese in a rectangular .25-inch layer over the plastic wrap, ensure that cream cheese has reached room temperature and been whipped until fluffy.

- Spread diced pickles over the cream cheese, then lay meats in overlapping layers over entirety.
- To flip the entire rectangle, add another layer of plastic wrap over meats and flip, then remove plastic from cream cheese side.
- Pull away the bottom layer of plastic wrap as you roll the rectangle into a tube shape.
- When the tube has been rolled, wrapped it tightly in plastic wrap, and added to the refrigerator for a minimum of 4 hours, slice it into 1-inch thick portions and keep refrigerated until ready to be consumed.

Note

These pinwheels may not freeze well and should be consumed within a couple of days.

No Bun Bacon Burger

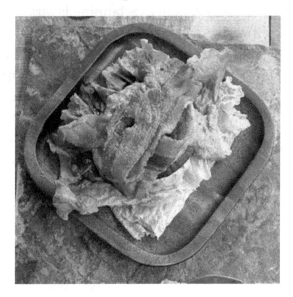

This recipe needs 30 minutes to prepare and makes 4 portions.

One portion size is 1 pattie; it contains:

68 grams Fat

54.4 grams Protein

8 grams Carbs

890 Calories

What's in It

Burger:
- Black Pepper (liberal sprinkle)
- Sea Salt (liberal sprinkle)
- Romaine Lettuce (8 leaves large)
- Red Onion (1 large)
- Bacon (8 slices)
- Pepper Jack Cheese (4 slices)
- Minced Beef (24 ounces)

Almond Butter Sauce:
- Rice Vinegar (1 tablespoon)
- Erythritol (1 teaspoon)
- Coconut Aminos (6 tablespoons)
- Thai Chili Peppers (4)
- Garlic (4 cloves peeled)
- Water (1 cup)
- Almond Butter (1 cup)

Also Needed:

- Broiling Pan
- Frying Pan
- Paper Towel
- Saucepan
- Food Processor

How It's Made

Burger:

- Ensure beef is thawed.
- Mold meat into 4 burgers before pressing the middle of each slightly around the center to ensure they do not form a ball during cooking.
- Add burgers to broiling pan before adding a liberal sprinkle of sea salt and black pepper.
- Add pan to a broiler that is set to a high temperature for a duration of 7 minutes before removing the pan and changing the orientation of the burgers, so the opposite side can cook.
- Add the pan to the broiler again for a duration of 7 minutes before removing the pan and adding cheese atop the burgers.
- Add the pan to the broiler for a duration of 5 minutes.
- Cut red onion into .25-inch slices.
- Add frying pan to a stove over a burner that is turned to a medium heat before adding bacon. Cook the bacon until crisp.
- Lay bacon on a paper towel to soak up the resulting grease.
- Add 2 leaves of lettuce to the bottom of each container before adding 1 burger and 1 cut of red onion to each container.
- Add bacon and almond butter sauce to each burger.

Almond Butter Sauce:

- Put a saucepan to a stove over a burner that is turned to a low heat before adding water and almond butter to the saucepan.
- Allow contents to come to a bubbling simmer and continue moving contents with a spoon until the contents become thick.
- Before adding coconut aminos to the contents, turn off the burner. Add and mix.
- Add erythritol, rice vinegar, Thai chili peppers and cloves of garlic to the food processor and mix until a paste is made.
- Add the paste to the contents of the saucepan and mix well.

Note

Store almond butter sauce, lettuce, and patties separately when freezing patties. This recipe can be changed a few ways. The patties can be fried in a skillet rather than baked. Cooked patties will freeze well, as will uncooked patties. Form the burgers and freeze them on parchment paper until the patties are solid. Then place the frozen patties in an airtight container until you are ready for them. For tips on storing and rewarming meat see here. Almond butter sauce can be added to a jar and refrigerated. Glass jars are ideal and easier to clean.

Vietnamese Meatballs

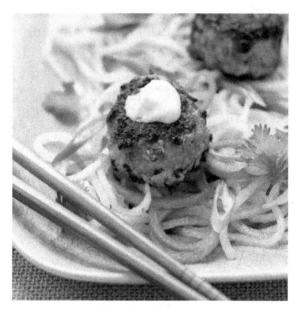

This recipe needs 1 hour to prepare and makes 4 portions.

One portion size is4 meatballs, .5 cups vegetables, 2 tablespoons mayonnaise; it contains:

45 grams Fat

25 grams Protein

6 grams Carbs

529 Calories

What's in It

Mayonnaise Sauce:
- Rice Vinegar (1 teaspoon)
- Erythritol (1 tablespoon)
- Sriracha (1 tablespoon)
- Mayonnaise (.5 cups)

Meatballs:
- Garlic Powder (.5 teaspoons)
- Salt (.25 teaspoons)
- Erythritol (1 tablespoon)
- Fish Sauce (2 tablespoons)
- Cilantro (2 tablespoons chopped)
- Scallions (.25 cups chopped)
- Ginger (1 teaspoon minced)
- Almond Flour (.25 cups)
- Eggs (1)
- Minced Pork (1 pound)

Pickled Vegetables:
- Fish Sauce (1 teaspoon)
- Erythritol (.25 cups)
- Rice Vinegar (.3 cups)
- Carrot (1 julienned)
- Medium Radish (1 julienned)

Also Needed:

- Mixing Bowl (3 medium, 1 small)
- Frying Pan

How It's Made

Mayonnaise Sauce:
- Add rice vinegar, erythritol, sriracha, and mayonnaise to a mixing bowl and blend well.

Meatballs:
- Add garlic powder, salt, erythritol, fish sauce, cilantro, scallions, ginger, almond flour, egg and pork to a mixing bowl and combine thoroughly.
- Divide contents into 16 meatballs.
- Add a pan to the stove above a burner that is turned to a medium heat before cooking meatballs until the outside is browned.

Pickled Vegetables:
- Add fish sauce, erythritol, and rice vinegar to a small bowl and whisk thoroughly.
- Add the carrot and radish to a medium bowl before pouring prepared sauce over the vegetables and ensuring they are well coated.

- Add the bowl of vegetables to the refrigerator for a duration of 1 hour, ensuring that the results are mixed with a spoon occasionally.

Note

Store pickled vegetables, mayonnaise sauce, and meatballs separately when freezing meatballs. This recipe can be changed a few ways. The meatballs can be baked rather than fried. Cooked meatballs will freeze well, as will uncooked meatballs. Form the meatballs and freeze them on parchment paper until the meatballs are solid. Then place the frozen meatballs in an airtight container until you are ready for them. For tips on storing and rewarming meat see here. Mayonnaise sauce should be added to the refrigerator in a glass jar. Pickled vegetables should be added to a refrigerator in a lidded bowl. More time in the refrigerator can ensure you end up with more flavorful pickled vegetables.

Tuna Zucchini Casserole

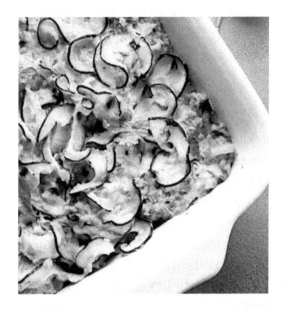

This recipe needs 30 minutes to prepare and makes 6.5 portions.

One portion size is .17 of total casserole; it contains:

16.1 grams Fat

10.3 grams Protein

6.6 grams Carbs

209 Calories

What's in It

- Red Pepper Flakes (.5 teaspoons)
- Coconut Milk (.5 cups)
- Coconut Flour (2 tablespoons)
- Avocado Oil (1 tablespoon)
- Celery (.5 cups chopped)
- Onion (.5 cup chopped)
- Black Pepper (.25 teaspoons)
- Garlic Powder (.25 teaspoons)
- Spicy Mustard (1 tablespoon)
- Seasoning Salt (.5 teaspoons)
- Chives (2 tablespoons chopped)
- Mayonnaise (.5 cups)
- Green Chiles (4 ounces diced)
- Canned Tuna (10 ounces)
- Zucchini (3)

Also Needed:

- Spiralizer
- Mixing Bowl (2)
- Frying Pan
- Casserole Dish (9 inches wide by 13 inches long)

How It's Made

- Ensure oven is heated to a temperature of 350 degrees Fahrenheit and the casserole dish is lightly oiled.
- Remove water from the can of tuna before adding tuna, garlic powder, black pepper, mustard, chives, green chiles, and mayonnaise to a mixing bowl and combining them well.
- Add oil to a pan before adding the pan to the stove above a burner that is turned to a medium heat.
- Add celery and onion to the pan to cook for a duration of approximately 6 minutes.
- Add coconut milk and coconut flour to the pan and mix the contents until no chunks are present.
- Spiralize zucchini and add them to a paper towel. Use this paper towel to press any excess water out of the zucchini.
- Add zucchini to the pan and mix. Allow the mix to cook for a duration of approximately 1.5 minutes.
- Take the pan away from the stove and add the contents to a large bowl.

- Add the contents of the bowl containing tuna to the bowl containing the pan contents and mix.
- Add the results to the casserole dish before adding the dish to the oven for a duration of 10 to 15 minutes.
- Allow the dish to cool thoroughly before adding to freezer.

Note

After being frozen and warmed, this casserole may have extra water. To see instructions on the proper way to store and reheat a casserole, click here.

Hamburger Casserole

This recipe needs 50 minutes to prepare and cook and makes 4 portions.

One portion size is .25 of total casserole; it contains:

26.8 grams Fat

39 grams Protein

16.2 grams Carbs

443 Calories

What's in It

- Almonds (.25 cups sliced)
- Eggs (2)
- Chicken Broth (1 cup)
- Coconut Milk (1 cup)
- Salt (to taste)
- Pepper (to taste)
- Dry Oregano (.5 teaspoons)
- Paprika (1 teaspoon)
- Cumin (1 teaspoon)
- Minced Beef (1 pound)
- Cauliflower (1 head)

Also Needed:

- Steamer Pot
- Frying Pan
- Casserole Dish

How It's Made

- Ensure the oven is preheated to a temperature of 350 degrees Fahrenheit.

- Cut the cauliflower florets away from the core before chopping the florets.
- Add a steamer pot to the stove above a burner that is turned to a medium heat.
- Before adding the cauliflower to the upper portion of the steamer pot, adding salt to the cauliflower, and covering the pot with a lid- add 2 inches of water to the bottom portion of the steamer pot.
- Allow the cauliflower to steam until it is barely cooked before taking it away from the heat.
- Add a pan to the stove above a burner that is turned to a medium heat before adding the minced beef, oregano, paprika, cumin, salt and pepper to the pan.
- With a spatula, break down the beef as it cooks so the pieces are very small.
- As the beef is nearing completion of cooking, take it away from the heat.
- Add broth, eggs, cream, salt, and pepper to a bowl and whip together.
- Add the cooked beef and cauliflower to the bottom of a casserole dish before pouring the egg combination over them.
- Add the casserole dish to the oven for a duration of 40 to 45 minutes.
- Take the casserole out of the oven before adding sliced almonds to the top.

- Add the casserole to the oven under a broiler for a duration of 2 to 3 minutes.
- Ensure the casserole has cooled thoroughly before adding it to a refrigerator or freezer.

Note

After being frozen and warmed, this casserole may have extra water. To see instructions on the proper way to store and reheat a casserole, <u>click here.</u>

Indian Inspired Sloppy Joes

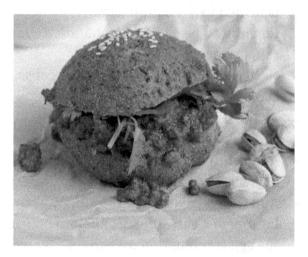

This recipe needs 30 minutes to prepare and makes 6 portions.

One portion size is 1 sandwich; it contains:

16.8 grams Fat

29.8 grams Protein

23.3 grams Carbs

366 Calories

What's in It

Keto Friendly Buns:
- Sesame Seeds (5 tablespoons)
- Sea Salt (1 teaspoon)
- Baking Soda (1 teaspoon)
- Cream of Tartar (2 tablespoons)
- Onion Powder (2 teaspoons)
- Garlic Powder (2 teaspoons)
- Flax Meal (.5 cups packed)
- Coconut Flour (.5 cups)
- Psyllium Husk (.3 cups powdered)
- Almond Flour (1.5 cups)
- Water (2 cups boiling)
- Eggs (2 whole, 6 whites)

Meat:
- Chili (1 crushed)
- Minced Turkey (1 pound)
- White Onion (.3 cups diced)
- Cumin Seeds (1 teaspoon)

- Avocado Oil (2 tablespoons)

Sauce:
- Paprika (.5 teaspoons)
- Sea Salt (1 teaspoon)
- Garam Masala (1 teaspoon)
- Chili (1 crushed)
- Water (.75 cups)
- Sugarless Tomato Sauce (15 ounces)
- Garlic (1 clove minced)
- Ginger (1 tablespoon minced)
- Avocado Oil (3 tablespoons)
- Pistachios (.25 cups shelled)
- Coconut Milk (.25 cups)
- Apple Cider Vinegar (1 teaspoon)
- Cilantro (.25 cups chopped)

Also Needed:

- Mixing Bowl
- Mixer
- Baking Pan
- Parchment Paper
- Frying Pan
- Saucepan

How It's Made

Keto Friendly Buns:

- Ensure the oven is preheated to a temperature of 350 degrees Fahrenheit and a baking pan is lined with parchment paper.
- Add salt, baking soda, cream of tartar, onion powder, garlic powder, psyllium husk powder, flax meal, coconut flour and almond flour to a mixing bowl and combine well before adding 2 whole eggs and only the whites of 6 eggs to the contents.
- Use a mixer and continue moving the contents until it becomes a thick dough.
- Before continuing to mix, add boiling water to the contents.
- Ensure the contents are well blended before separating the dough into 10 balls and adding them to the baking pan.
- Drop sesame seeds in a thin layer atop each ball of dough before gently pressing the seeds into the dough.
- Add the baking pan to the oven for a duration of 45 to 50 minutes.
- Ensure the buns are cooled thoroughly before slicing and freezing.

Meat and Sauce:
- Add a pan to the stove above a burner that is turned to a medium to low heat before adding 1 tablespoon of avocado oil and the

pistachios to cook for a duration of 4 to 5 minutes then be removed.

- Add a saucepan to the stove above a burner that is turned to a medium heat before adding garlic, ginger, and 2 tablespoons of avocado oil to the pan to cook for a duration of 1 minute.
- Add paprika, salt, garam masala, chili, water, and tomato sauce to the pan before adding a lid to the pan and boiling the contents.
- Turn down the burner under the pan to a low heat when the contents begin to bubble to allow the sauce to simmer.
- Add the frying pan to the stove above a burner turned to a medium to low heat before adding cumin seeds and 2 tablespoons of avocado oil to cook for a duration of 1 minute.
- Add onion to the pan to cook for a duration of 5 minutes before adding the chili and turkey to continue cooking until cooked thoroughly.
- Before increasing the heat of the burner under the saucepan to a medium heat, add the cooked meat to the sauce contents.
- Allow the combined contents to heat until bubbling before turning the burner to a low heat to simmer for a duration of 15 minutes.

Ensure the steam has been released from under the lid before turning down the heat.

- Add pistachios, apple cider vinegar, and coconut milk to the contents of the saucepan.
- Ensure the mixture has cooled thoroughly before adding the results to a freezer.

Note

This meat mixture will freeze and thaw well. It should be consumed within 2 months. Store bread and meat separately. This bread recipe can be used to make buns that will be used for other low-carb sandwiches or meals. To see instructions of freezing and usage of meat-based meals click here. To see instruction on freezing and usage of bread see here.

Turkey and Vegetable Stew

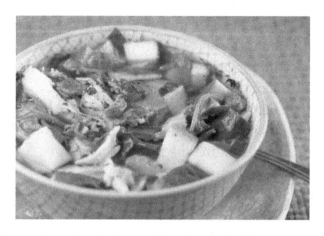

This recipe needs 40 minutes to prepare and cook and makes 4 portions.

One portion size is 1 bowl; it contains:

23.6 grams Fat

46 grams Protein

13.1 grams Carbs

449 Calories

What's in It

- Black Pepper (.13 teaspoons)
- Sea Salt (.13 teaspoons)
- Turkey Breast (12 ounces)
- Water (2 cups)
- Chicken Broth (4 cups)

- Tomatoes (3 diced)
- Baby Spinach (4 cups)
- Zucchini (2 diced)
- Italian Seasoning (1 tablespoon)
- Garlic (2 cloves minced)
- Celery (2 stalks diced)
- Onion (1 diced)
- Bacon (12 slices diced)

Also Needed:

- Pot

How It's Made

- Add a pot to the stove above a burner that is turned to a medium heat before adding celery, onion, and bacon to the pot to cook until the vegetables soften and the bacon browns.
- Add zucchini, pepper, salt, Italian seasoning, and garlic to the pot to cook for a duration of 1 minute before adding tomatoes and spinach to the contents of the pot and stirring until the spinach has wilted.
- Add water and broth to the pot and allow the contents to boil before adding the turkey breast to the pot.

- Turn the heat of the burner under the pot to a low heat and allowing the contents to simmer for a duration of 20 to 25 minutes before taking the turkey out of the pot and shredding it.
- Add the shredded turkey to the contents of the pot and mix.
- Allow the results to cool thoroughly before adding to a freezer.

Note

This soup should freeze and rewarm well. If you intend to freeze this soup, leave the vegetables slightly less cooked than you want them to be when you are ready to consume the soup. To see instructions on the proper way to store and reheat a soup, click here.

Sweet and Sour Pork

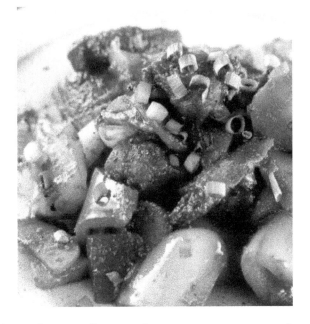

This recipe needs 25 minutes to prepare and cook and makes 4 portions.

One portion size is .25 of total; it contains:

39.8 grams Fat

43.12 grams Protein

15.94 grams Carbs

598 Calories

What's in It

Sweet and Sour Sauce:

- Stevia Powder (.25 teaspoons)
- Granulated Chicken Stock (1 teaspoons)
- White Vinegar (4 tablespoons)
- Coconut Aminos (4 tablespoons)
- Tomato Paste (4 tablespoons)

Meat:

- Olive Oil (6 tablespoons)
- Coconut Flour (1 tablespoons)
- Black Pepper (1 teaspoons)
- Salt (1 teaspoons)
- Pork Roast (21 ounces cut into pieces)
- Onion (1 diced)
- Carrot (.5 thinly sliced)
- Red Pepper (1 chopped)
- Yellow Pepper (1 chopped)

Also Needed:

- Small Bowl
- Frying Pan

How It's Made

- Add stevia powder, granulated chicken stock, white vinegar, coconut aminos, and tomato paste to a small bowl and mix well.
- Coat the pork with coconut flour, pepper, and salt.

- Add a frying pan to the stove above a burner that is turned to a medium heat before adding the pork and 4 tablespoons olive oil to the pan.
- Take the pork out of the pan before adding onion, carrot, red pepper, yellow pepper, and 2 tablespoon of olive oil to the pan.
- Allow the vegetables to cook until they begin to soften before adding the pork to the pan and mixing.
- Add the sauce to the contents of the pan and cook the contents for a duration of 1 minute.
- Allow the results to fully cool before adding to a refrigerator or freezer.

Note

Add the sauce to a refrigerator independent of the other contents which may be added to a freezer. Ensure that you are aware of the correct way to reheat meals with ingredients that warm at different rates. To see more about what this entails, click here.

Chile Cheese Burgers

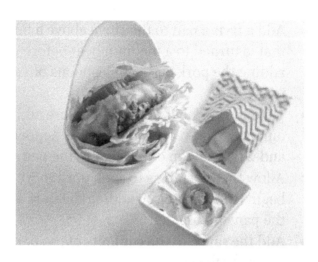

This recipe needs 15 minutes to prepare and cook and makes 4 portions.

One portion size is 1 burger; it contains:

37.2 grams Fat

26 grams Protein

1.8 grams Carbs

450 Calories

What's in It

- Mayonnaise (4 tablespoons)
- Canned Green Chiles (4 ounces drained and diced)
- Garlic (1 clove minced)

- Colby Jack Cheese (4 slices)
- Salt (.13 teaspoons)
- Black Pepper (.13 teaspoons)
- Coconut Oil (1 tablespoon)
- Hot Sauce (1 teaspoon)
- Cumin (.75 tablespoons)
- Chili Powder (.25 teaspoons)
- Red Onion (4 slices)
- Minced Beef (1 pound)

Also Needed:

- Mixing Bowl (1 large 1 small)
- Frying Pan

How It's Made

- Add green chiles, hot sauce, garlic, chili powder, and .25 tablespoons of cumin to beef in a large bowl.
- Combine contents thoroughly before separating the results into 4 burger patties.
- Add a frying pan to the stove above a burner that is turned to a medium heat before adding coconut oil and patties to fry until patties are sufficiently cooked.
- Add .5 tablespoons of cumin to mayonnaise in a small bowl and mix well.
- Store mayonnaise and burgers separately until ready to consume.

Note

This recipe can be changed a few ways. The patties can be baked rather than being fried in a skillet. Cooked patties will freeze well, as will uncooked patties. Form the burgers and freeze them on parchment paper until the patties are solid. Then place the frozen patties in an airtight container until you are ready for them. For tips on storing and rewarming meat see here. These burger patties can be wrapped with lettuce or served on the Keto Buns from another recipe.

Bacon Wrapped Chicken Pepper Bites

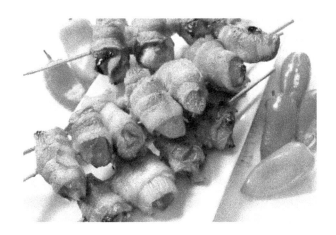

This recipe needs 45 minutes to prepare and makes 4 portions.

One portion size is 1 skewer; it contains:

28 grams Fat

64 grams Protein

1 grams Carbs

533 Calories

What's in It

- Black Pepper (.13 teaspoons)
- Sea Salt (.5 teaspoons)
- Paprika (1 teaspoon)
- Bacon (.5 pounds)
- Sweet Peppers (16)

- Boneless Chicken (2 pounds cut into small pieces)

Also Needed:

- Wooden Skewers

How It's Made

- Ensure the oven is heated to a temperature of 425 degrees Fahrenheit.
- Add black pepper, sea salt, and paprika to chicken pieces.
- Take the stems off of the peppers with a knife and cut an opening along the pepper to remove the seeds before cutting bacon strips in half to make shorter strips.
- Add one piece of chicken to the inside of each pepper before wrapping each pepper with a piece of bacon and poking a wooden skewer through the wrapped pepper.
- Keep following this routine until all peppers are stuffed and skewered. Allow 4 to 6 peppers on each skewer.
- Add the skewers to the oven for a duration of 35 minutes.
- Allow results to cool thoroughly before adding to a refrigerator or freezer.

Note

These bites can be frozen while still on the wooden skewers. For tips on storing and rewarming meat see here.

Chapter 5: Keto Dinner Recipes

A collection of hearties, Keto approved meals to satisfy the whole household. These recipes can be used for lunches as well. High in healthy fat, low in carbohydrates, and easy to prepare on meal prep day and enjoy for meals to come.

Chicken Enchilada Bowl

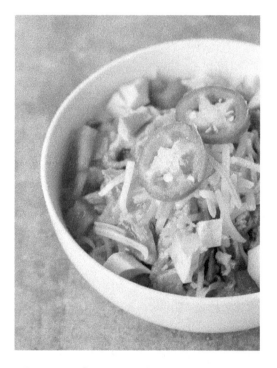

This recipe needs 30 minutes to prepare and makes 4 portions.

One portion size is 1 bowl; it contains:

2 grams Fat

18 grams Protein

6 grams Carbs

120 Calories

What's in It

- Avocado (.5 sliced)
- Cheese (.25 cup)
- Olive Oil (1 tablespoon)
- Riced Cauliflower (12 ounces steamed)
- Green Chiles (4 ounces canned)
- Onion (.25 cups)
- Water (.25 cups)
- Red Enchilada Sauce (.75 cups)
- Chicken Breasts (1 pound)

Also Needed:

- Frying Pan (2)

How It's Made

- Before you add the pan to the stove over a burner turned to a medium heat to lightly brown the chicken breasts, cut the meat into 4 large pieces.

- Add water, onions, chiles, and sauce to the pan and allow it all to simmer under a lid until the chicken is cooked through (a duration of approximately 25 minutes).
- Once the cooked chicken has been removed from the pan and shredded, add it to the same pan and simmer until the juices have been mostly absorbed (a duration of approximately 10 minutes).
- Add another pan to the stove above a burner turned to medium heat and saute cauliflower with 1 tablespoon of oil for a duration of 5 to 7 minutes.
- After the food has a chance to cook, separate rice and enchilada chicken into 4 lidded containers, add avocado and cheese, then refrigerate until ready to be consumed.

Note

These pre-portioned meals can be added to the freezer. If you choose to freeze these meals, add the avocado to a refrigerator separate to the rest of the meal and combine when ready to be consumed. To find tips on reheating meals that contain foods that rewarm differently, click here.

Steak Bits

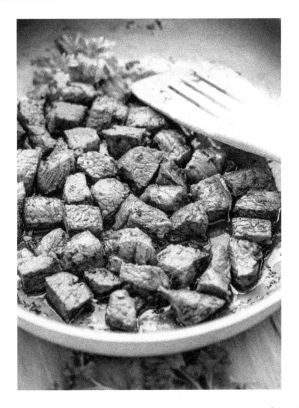

This recipe needs 15 minutes to prepare and makes 4 portions.

One portion size is 6 ounces; it contains:

48.8 grams Fat

36.7 grams Protein

11.5 grams Carbs

629 Calories

What's 1in It

- Top Sirloin Steak (24 ounces)
- Black Pepper (1 teaspoon)
- Parsley (1 tablespoon dry)
- Basil (2 tablespoons dry)
- Garlic (1 teaspoon minced)
- Worcestershire Sauce (.25 cups)
- Olive Oil (.3 cups)
- Soy Sauce (.5 cups)

Also Needed:

- Plastic Ziplock Bag
- Frying Pan

How It's Made

- Ensure that steak is sliced into 1-inch pieces before adding all ingredients to a large plastic ziplock bag and stirring with a spoon. If you'd like to allow the meat to marinate, add to the refrigerator for a duration of 3 hours. If not, shake the bag to coat the meat with marinade.
- Add a pan to the stove above a burner turned to medium/high heat and let sit

until hot then cook the meat pieces. Throw away the extra marinade.

- Allow meat to cool once it is cooked and separate the results into 4 portions to add to refrigerator or freezer until ready to be consumed.

Note

Allowing the meat to marinate for a duration of 3 hours or longer will improve the flavor of the dish. Meat pieces can be frozen cooked or be frozen in the marinade. To see tips on freezing and rewarming meats, click here.

Sausage and Bacon Meatballs

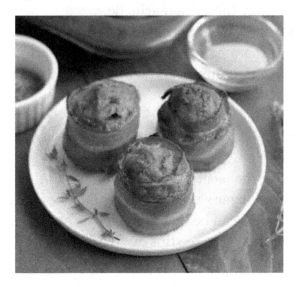

This recipe needs 40 minutes to prepare and makes 9 portions.

One portion size is 1 meatball; it contains:

7 grams Fat

12 grams Protein

2 grams Carbs

What's in It

- Oregano (1 tablespoon dried)
- White Onion (2 tablespoons diced)
- Garlic (2 tablespoons minced)
- Sugar-Free Bacon (9 slices)
- Spicy Italian Sausage (1 pound)

Also Needed:

- Muffin Tin (9 sections)

How It's Made

- Ensure that the oven is preheated to a temperature of 375 degrees Fahrenheit and a muffin tin is lightly oiled with coconut oil.
- Add the oregano, onion, sausage, and garlic to a large bowl and mix.
- Separate the mixture into 9 equal balls and wrap one slice of bacon around each.
- Add the wrapped meatballs to the oiled muffin tin and add to the oven for a duration of 30 minutes followed by broiling for a duration of 5 minutes.
- Separate resulting portions into containers once cooled and add to refrigerator or freezer until ready to be consumed.

Note

This recipe can be changed a few ways. The meatballs can be added to a frying pan rather than baked. Cooked meatballs will freeze well, as will uncooked meatballs. Form the meatballs and freeze them on parchment paper until the meatballs are solid. Then place the frozen meatballs in an airtight container until you are ready for them. For tips on storing and rewarming meat see here.

Chicken Fajitas

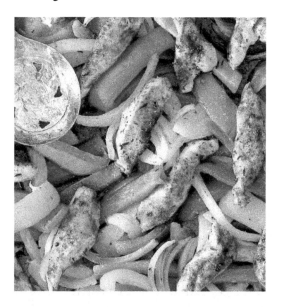

This recipe needs 35 minutes to prepare and makes 4 portions.

One portion size is 1 bowl; it contains:

7.12 grams Fat

30 grams Protein

14.1 grams Carbs

244 Calories

What's in It

- Riced Cauliflower (12 ounces)
- Lime (1 sliced)
- Yellow Onion (1 medium sliced thin)
- Red Bell Pepper (3 medium sliced)
- Taco Seasoning (1 tablespoon)
- Chicken Breast (24 ounces)
- Olive Oil (3 tablespoons)

Also Needed:

- Baking Pan

How It's Made

- Ensure that the oven is preheated to a temperature of 400 degrees Fahrenheit and a baking pan is oiled lightly.

- Before coating the chicken with seasoning, cut the meat into strips. Trickle olive oil over the coated chicken.
- Before adding chicken and vegetables to the pan, cut the onion and peppers into slices.
- Add the pan to the oven for a duration of 20 to 25 minutes before taking it out and dribbling juice from the lime onto the results.
- Add a skillet to the stove above a burner turned to medium heat and saute cauliflower with 1 tablespoon of oil for a duration of 5 to 7 minutes.
- Separate results into 4 containers once cooled and add to refrigerator or freezer until ready to eat.

Note

In instances like this, the foods that are stored together in a meal prep container will reheat using different ideal durations and temperatures. To see tips on heating meals with different ingredients, click here.

Pizza Style Chicken Breast

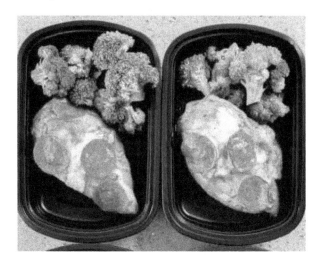

This recipe needs 26 minutes to prepare and makes 4 portions.

One portion size is 1 chicken breast and .5 cups broccoli; it contains:

15 grams Fat

35 grams Protein

8 grams Carbs

What's in It

- Broccoli (2 cups cut into florets)
- Pepperoni (2 ounces)

- Mozzarella (4 ounces)
- Pizza Seasoning (1.5 tablespoons)
- Pizza Sauce (.5 cups)
- Chicken Breast (1 pound)

Also Needed:

- Baking Sheet

How It's Made

- Ensure that the oven is preheated to a temperature of 375 degrees Fahrenheit and chicken breasts are placed on a baking sheet. Add pizza seasoning and sauce over top of chicken breasts.
- Add the baking sheet to the oven for a duration of 8 to 10 minutes before removing and topping with mozzarella, then again add to the oven for a duration of 6 minutes.
- Add pepperoni atop the chicken breasts and add to the oven until the chicken's internal temperature reaches a temperature of 165 degrees Fahrenheit.
- Add broccoli to a lidded, microwave-safe dish with 2 tablespoons of water and microwave on high for a duration of 4 minutes.

- Separate resulting broccoli and chicken into 4 lidded containers and add to refrigerator or freezer until ready to consume.

Note

In instances like this, the foods that are stored together in a meal prep container will reheat using different ideal durations and temperatures. To see tips on heating meals with different ingredients, click here. To see tips on storing and reheating meats, click here.

Low Carb Chili

This recipe needs 40 minutes to prepare and makes 6 portions.

One portion size is 1 cup; it contains:

5.5 grams Fat

24.3 grams Protein

7.3 grams Carbs

178 Calories

What's in It

- Onion Powder (2 teaspoons)
- Garlic Powder (1 teaspoon)
- Cumin Powder (1 tablespoon)
- Cayenne Pepper (.5 teaspoons)
- Chili Powder (2 tablespoons)
- Sea Salt (1.5 teaspoons)
- Water (1 cup)
- Cherry Tomatoes (1 cup chopped)
- Crushed Tomatoes (28 ounces)
- Medium Onion (1 chopped)
- Olive Oil (1 tablespoon)
- Garlic (2 cloves crushed)
- Minced Beef (1 pound)

Also Needed:

- Large Pot

How It's Made

- Add a pot to the stove above a burner that is turned to a medium to high heat before adding olive oil, garlic, onion and beef and cooking until beef is browned.
- Add salt, chili powder, cayenne pepper, cumin powder, garlic powder, onion powder, water, crushed tomatoes and cherry tomatoes to the pot and stir.

- Cook until the contents are bubbling, then bring the heat of the burner down to a medium to low heat and continue cooking for a duration of 30 minutes.
- Ensure results have cooled before adding to the refrigerator or freezer for later consumption.

Note

This chili should freeze and rewarm well. When rewarming, you can add more crushed tomatoes to maintain the texture of the chili. Be aware that this will change the nutritional value of each serving. To see instructions on the proper way to store and reheat a soup, click here.

Thai Chicken Soup

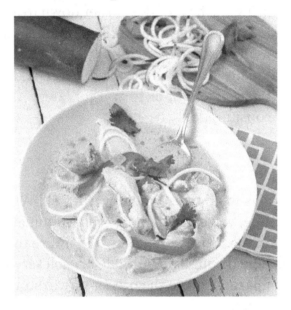

This recipe needs 30 minutes to prepare and makes 8 portions.

One portion size is 1 cup; it contains:

14.92 grams Fat

24.42 grams Protein

8.91 grams Carbs

271 Calories

What's in It

- Lime (1 sliced)
- Zucchini (2 spiralized)
- Cilantro (.5 cups chopped)
- Fish Sauce (2 tablespoons)
- Chicken Breast (1 pound sliced thin)
- Red Pepper (1 sliced thin)
- Coconut Milk (15 ounces)
- Chicken Bone Broth (6 cups)
- Garlic (2 cloves minced)
- Green Curry Paste (1.5 tablespoons)
- Jalapeno (1 chopped)
- Onion (.5 chopped)
- Coconut Oil (1 tablespoon)

Also Needed:

- Spiralizer
- Pot

How It's Made

- Add a pot to the stove above a burner that is turned to a medium heat before adding the onion and coconut oil and cooking for a duration of approximately 5 minutes until the onions become slightly see-through.
- Add garlic, green curry paste, and jalapeno to the onion and cook for a duration of 1

minute before adding the coconut milk and chicken broth to the pot and mixing well.

- Ensure that the contents reach a boil before turning down the heat under the burner to medium.
- Add fish sauce, chicken, and red pepper to the pot before simmering for a duration of 5 to 7 minutes.
- Add cilantro to the pot.
- Make zucchini pasta using a spiralizer.
- Store zucchini pasta, soup, and lime separately. Add together when ready to be consumed.

Note

This soup should freeze and rewarm well. If you intend to freeze this soup, leave the vegetables slightly less cooked than you want them to be when you are ready to consume the soup. To see instructions on the proper way to store and reheat a soup, click here.

Broccoli Cheese Soup

This recipe needs 30 minutes to prepare and makes 4 portions.

One portion size is 1 cup; it contains:

52.3 grams Fat

23.85 grams Protein

9.88 grams Carbs

561 Calories

What's in It

- Heavy Cream (.75 cup)
- Salt (to taste)
- Black Pepper (to taste)
- Sharp Cheddar Cheese (3 cups shredded)
- Garlic (1 teaspoon minced)
- Vegetable Stock (1.5 cups)
- Broccoli (4 cups chopped)
- Small Onion (1 diced)

Also Needed:

- Pot

How It's Made

- Add a pot to the stove above a burner that is turned to a medium heat before adding the onion, garlic, and broccoli to cook for a duration of around 5 minutes.

- Allow the contents to boil before placing a lid on the pot and turning down the heat to simmer for a duration of 10 minutes.
- Add the heavy cream to the pot and allow to cook for a duration of 3 to 5 minutes.
- Add the cheese to the pot and stir until velvety and well mixed. This will take a duration of approximately 1 to 2 minutes.
- Once cooled, store entire soup as one or separate into portions.

Note

This soup should freeze and rewarm well. If you intend to freeze this soup, know that soups containing dairy need a longer duration of time to reheat because the dairy products could begin to curdle. To see instructions on the proper way to store and reheat soup, click here.

Pork and Pepper Stew

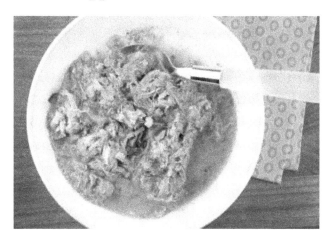

This recipe needs 3 hours to prepare and makes 4 portions.

One portion size is 1 bowl; it contains:

36.2 grams Fat

37 grams Protein

8.9 grams Carbs

515 Calories

What's in It

- Black Pepper (.13 teaspoons)
- Sea Salt (.13 teaspoons)
- Basil (.5 cups chopped)

- Lime (1 juiced)
- Tomato Paste (3 tablespoons)
- Chicken Broth (4 cups)
- Garlic (3 cloves minced)
- Cumin Seeds (.5 teaspoons)
- Chili Powder (1 teaspoon)
- Onion (1 diced)
- Jalapeno (2 seeded and diced)
- Yellow Pepper (1 seeded and diced)
- Red Pepper (1 seeded and diced)
- Pork Roast (2 pounds cut into pieces)
- Olive Oil (2 tablespoons)

Also Needed:

- Pot

How It's Made

- Add a pot to the stove above a burner that is turned to a medium heat before adding the pork and olive oil and cooking the meat until browned before removing.
- Add the onions and peppers to the pot to cook until they begin to soften.
- Add garlic, cumin, and chili powder to the vegetables to cook for a duration of 1 minute before adding the pork to the pan.
- Add tomato paste and chicken broth to the pan and allow the contents to heat bubbling

before turning down the heat of the burner under the pan to low heat and allowing the contents to simmer for a duration of 2 hours.

- Remove the pork from the pan and shred it before adding it back to the contents of the pan.
- Ensure the results have cooled thoroughly before adding the stew to a refrigerator or freezer.

Note

This soup should freeze and rewarm well. If you intend to freeze this soup, leave the vegetables slightly less cooked than you want them to be when you are ready to consume the soup. To see instructions on the proper way to store and reheat soup, click here.

Cabbage Lasagna

This recipe needs 45 minutes to prepare and makes 20 portions.

One portion size is 379 grams; it contains:

34 grams Fat

27 grams Protein

9 grams Carbs

451 Calories

What's in It

- Mozzarella Cheese (32 ounces shredded)
- Sugarless Marinara Sauce (40 ounces)
- Minced Beef (2 pounds)
- Eggs (3)
- Dry Parsley (.25 cups)
- Parmesan Cheese (1.5 cups)
- Ricotta Cheese (3 pounds)
- Cabbage (1 head)
- Salt (1 teaspoon)

Also Needed:

- Pot
- Mixing Bowl
- Large Frying Pan
- Baking Pan (11 inches wide and 15 inches long)

How It's Made

- Ensure the oven is heated to a temperature of 350 degrees fahrenheit.

- Add a pot that is filled halfway with water to the stove above a burner turned to a high head before adding salt to the water and placing leaves of cabbage into the water to boil for a duration of 5 to 10 minutes.
- Take the cabbage out of the water and use a paper towel to remove any excess water.
- Add eggs, parsley, parmesan cheese and ricotta cheese to a bowl and mix well.
- Add a frying pan to the stove above a burner that is set to a medium to high heat before adding meat to the pan and cooking until it is brown.
- Add marinara sauce to the meat.
- Add .75 cups of meat sauce to the bottom of the baking pan.
- Lay 1 layer of cabbage leaves over the sauce in the baking pan, so the sauce is covered.
- Add the cheese mixture atop the cabbage leaf layer.
- Add half of the meat sauce atop the cheese layer.
- Add a layer of mozzarella cheese atop the new sauce layer.
- Copy the same layering steps until all of the ingredients have been used.
- Add the baking pan to the oven for a duration of 25 minutes.

- Ensure the food has cooled thoroughly before adding to the freezer or refrigerator.

Note

After being frozen and warmed, this lasagna may have extra water due to the cabbage. To see instructions on the proper way to store and reheat a casserole, click here.

BONUS RECIPE

Cloud bread is named for its appearance and is a keto staple. Many methods are available, but some have a tendency to have an odd texture. This recipe variation makes a great option for the days when bread cravings hit.

Cloud Bread

This recipe needs 65 minutes to prepare and makes 1 loaf.

One portion size is 1 slice; it contains:

4.5 grams Fat

7.5 grams Protein

0.8 grams Carbs

84 Calories

What's in It

- Whey Protein Powder (.5 cups)
- Salt (.25 teaspoons)
- Onion Powder (.25 teaspoons)
- Garlic Powder (.25 teaspoons)
- Baking Powder (.5 teaspoons)
- Sour Cream (6 ounces)

- Cream of Tartar (.5 teaspoons)
- Eggs (6 separated)

Also Needed:

- Mixing Bowl
- Mixing Bowl
- Mixer
- Loaf Pan

How It's Made

- Ensure the oven is preheated to a temperature of 300 degrees Fahrenheit and a loaf pan is lightly greased.
- Add the whites of 6 eggs to a mixing bowl and whip until they become stiff.
- Add the yolks of 6 eggs to a separate bowl before adding protein powder, salt, onion powder, garlic powder, baking powder, sour cream, and cream of tartar and mixing well.
- Add the whipped whites of the eggs to the bowl containing the remaining contents in small doses. Fold a small portion of the whites into the contents and continue to add the whites in small portions until the two bowls are fully combined.
- Add the mixture to a loaf pan before adding the loaf pan to the middle shelf of the oven for a duration of 50 to 60 minutes. When a

toothpick can be stabbed gently into the middle of the pan and pulled out without retaining any of the bread on it, the loaf is cooked.

- Ensure the bread has cooled thoroughly before cutting it into slices.

Note

This bread should be kept refrigerated. For best texture, add bread slices to a toaster before consuming. This recipe can be used to make rolls if desired. 18 rolls can be made from this dough. Be aware that the portion size would then change, and the nutrition information may change as well. The recipe will stay the same, but the cooking time will be altered from a duration of 50 to 60 minutes to a duration of 20 to 30 minutes.

Index for the Recipes

Chapter 3: Keto Breakfast Recipes

1. Chicken Maple Sausage Rounds
2. Avocado Shake
3. Keto Friendly Toast and Sugarless Jam
4. Keto Bagels
5. Omelette Bake
6. Keto Coffee
7. Chia and Coconut Bars
8. Spinach and Bacon Frittata
9. Cheesy Ham and Broccoli Egg Muffins
10. Stuffed Breakfast Biscuits

Chapter 4: Keto Lunch Recipes

1. Pinwheels
2. No Bun Bacon Burger
3. Vietnamese Meatballs
4. Tuna Zucchini Casserole
5. Hamburger Casserole
6. Indian Inspired Sloppy Joes
7. Turkey and Vegetable Stew
8. Sweet and Sour Pork
9. Chile Cheese Burgers
10. Bacon Wrapped Chicken Pepper Bites

Chapter 5: Keto Dinner Recipes

1. Enchilada Chicken Bowls
2. Steak Bits
3. Sausage and Bacon Meatballs
4. Chicken Fajitas
5. Pizza Style Chicken Breast
6. Low Carb Chili
7. Thai Chicken Soup
8. Broccoli Cheese Soup
9. Pork and Pepper Stew
10. Cabbage Lasagna

Bonus Recipe

11. Cloud Bread

Conclusion

I hope you enjoyed your copy of *Meal Prep for the Keto Diet*. Let's hope it was informative and provided you with the necessary tools to start saving time and decreasing stress by incorporating meal prep into your busy life.

The next step is to get prepping! Now you know how to plan for the week, store food properly and keep it in optimal condition when you're ready to eat. Your health and weight loss goals are important, and the goal of this book is to give you a resource to make them more attainable. Taking inspiration from various cuisines, this collection of scrumptious recipes has been compiled to broaden the horizons of your keto diet, so when your next meal prep day comes around you can pick a few recipes that inspire you and give them a try! Whether you are cooking for just yourself or feeding friends and family, there's a recipe for everyone and each food can be customized to fit your flavor needs. Have fun with your food.

Once your body reaches a state of ketosis, eating certain foods can bring it out of that state. This is why maintaining your Keto diet is important to achieve the results you are looking for. The Keto diet contains a specific type of food, and it can be difficult to find meals at restaurants or shops to suit your needs. Along the same vein, it can be difficult to be certain of the nutritional content in what you're consuming. Preparing your own food will give you peace of mind in knowing that you are able to follow your meal plan and get the results you want.

Finally, if you found this book useful in any way, a review on Amazon is always appreciated!

CPSIA information can be obtained
at www.ICGtesting.com
Printed in the USA
LVHW080925290719
625677LV00027B/313/P